Warming-Up

Your 6-Step Guide to the Perfect Dynamic Warm-Up

By PROSENCE

Copyright 2017 by Prosence - All rights reserved.

This document is geared towards providing exact and reliable information in regards to the topic and issue covered. The publication is sold with the idea that the publisher is not required to render accounting, officially permitted, or otherwise, qualified services. If advice is necessary, legal or professional, a practiced individual in the profession should be ordered.

- From a Declaration of Principles which was accepted and approved equally by a Committee of the American Bar Association and a Committee of Publishers and Associations.

The information provided herein is stated to be truthful and consistent, in that any liability, in terms of inattention or otherwise, by any usage or abuse of any policies, processes, or directions contained within is the solitary and utter responsibility of the recipient reader. Under no circumstances will any legal responsibility or blame be held against the publisher for any reparation, damages, or monetary loss due to the information herein, either directly or indirectly.

ABOUT PROSENCE

Our Mission

We are dedicated to guiding, motivating and providing the tools necessary to transform people into the best version of themselves. Our goal is to empower men and women across the globe to realize that physical and mental fitness are not a short-term solution, but a lifetime choice, and to actualize what they have come to understand into a daily routine. We invite you to discover this process for yourself as you join us in the exploration of science-based knowledge that can lead to better health, greater fulfillment and astonishing vitality.

Who is Prosence?

Prosence is led by Antonio Mazzotta, a strapping 28-year-old Italian health enthusiast who resides in Switzerland. He's a self-described "Mr. Nice Guy" who, (despite a powerful love for his mamma's pasta and pizza), has developed a life dedicated to health and fitness. Now, he strives to share his secrets with the world.

Antonio discovered his passion for health and fitness 7 years ago and has never looked back! Days are filled with working new routines at his gym, training hard, meeting like-minded people and, dear to his heart, teaching weight training, dieting, and healthy lifestyle choices to his valued clients. Job one is helping people to achieve their overall fitness goals, including providing a gain in endurance and a new (sustainable) vitality.

He and his team fight to counter the preponderance of bad information that proliferates the Internet, being driven by offering people a safe yet powerful path to vibrant, brilliant health. In short, Prosence is fervently dedicated to the motivation, inspiration and education of people via the dissemination of the real science-based information they need to get into great shape and to stay healthy for a lifetime.

Discover today how we can help you to grow into what you were meant to be and to embrace life to the fullest with newly realized passion!

Learn more on our website: www.prosencefitness.com, blog and keep up with the daily education and motivation by liking us on Twitter, Facebook & Instagram @prosence.

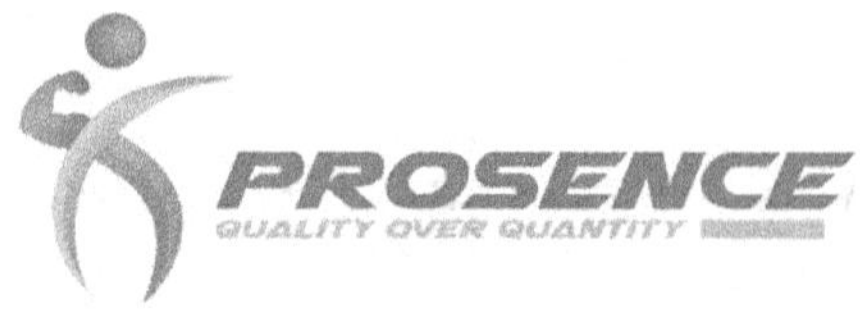

Table of Contents

Introduction

The way you start an exercise session greatly determines how you perform and the results you can get from it. Warming up before the main exercise session is the best way to prep yourself up for success in each and every exercise or workout session. But what's the best way to go about it?

In this book, you'll learn what dynamic warm ups are, why they are important, and more importantly, what makes for a very effective dynamic warm up routine, i.e., its structure. By the end of the book, you'll be in a great position to not just practice dynamic warm ups during your exercise sessions but also to come up with your very own dynamic warm up routine.

So if you're ready, turn the page and let's begin!

Chapter 1

The Importance of Warming Up

Many people are too busy trying to exercise right away that they forget to – or outright skip – the warming up process. Regardless of whether it's unintentional or intentional, the fact remains that warming up should never be neglected for many good reasons:

- It facilitates a less painful and easier movement through joint lubrication prior to the main exercises;

- It helps bring about hormonal production changes that can help your body use energy more efficiently;

- It helps improve nutrient and oxygen delivery to the muscles that'll be worked out, and this helps minimize your risks of getting tired or winded to easily or prematurely;

- It helps improve your reaction and coordination times;

- It helps increase blood flow to the muscles that'll be exercised, which prepares them much better for the upcoming workload;

- It helps minimize your risks for soft tissue injuries (muscles, tendons, and ligaments) by letting your joints and muscles move along a wider range of motion in a safer and easier manner;

- It helps raise your body's blood temperature and that can help you extend your workout times and put more effort into them;

- It helps to gradually prep your cardiovascular system, i.e., heart and lungs, for the strenuous activity that's to come, which will minimize your risk of a sudden spike in blood pressure;

- It helps you elevate the quality of your exercise sessions by priming up your body's nerve-muscle pathways for exercise; and

- It helps you prepare mentally for the upcoming workout, i.e., it helps you get all stoked up prior to exercising.

Dynamic Warm Ups Vs. Static Stretching

For the longest time, many sports performance professionals and experts have been looking for the best methods to help their clients achieve optimal performance. Given all things equal, people who are more physically conditioned, faster, stronger, and bigger tend to record the best physical performances during exercise and competition. While there's much debate as to the extent by which these factors affect physical performance during exercise or competitions, there's little disagreement as to the big contribution a comprehensive warm up session has in terms of peak performance with each and every exercise or workout session. That being said, is there an optimal way to warm up prior to exercising?

For the most part, people believe that the best way to prime up the body in preparation for a workout or exercise session is through a very light warm up followed by extensive static stretching. If you took the time to observe most people who exercise, you would find that they do a round or two of light jogs followed by a lot of static stretching. But this isn't the best way to go about warming the body up for a serious exercise or workout session.

When it comes to warming up, there are 2 ways many people do it: static stretching and dynamic warm ups. Static stretching is holding a specific stretching position for about 30 seconds to 1 minute, which is ideal for flexibility. Dynamic warm ups on the other hand, are based on movements that allow for loosening of the joints and to some extent, muscle stretching. Between the two, you must prioritize dynamic stretching. Why?

This is because dynamic stretching focuses on loosening your joints and muscles safely just before your workout. It's best to start with movements that are controlled and slow, which lets your upper and lower body move through a safe range or motion. After several slow-movement warm up exercises, you'll then move on to more upbeat and faster movements. It's been shown that performing dynamic warm-ups just before an exercise session can help increase your explosiveness, power, and total performance compared to merely static stretching.

If you focus more on doing dynamic warm ups or stretches, do more whole body movements and movements that involve stability. Never over stretch any joint or muscle while doing so. Remember the point of warming up in general is to minimize risks for injuries and not increase them. You must've broken a sweat, warmed up your muscles, and raised your blood pressure by the time your warm up's over.

Static stretches are fine for as long as your muscles have already been warmed up or loosened up. Otherwise, stretching muscles that are still tense and cold may result in muscle injuries like strains or worse, tears. That's why if you're going to incorporate it into your exercise program, it'll be much better to either put it at the end of your warm ups or after the exercise as part of the cool down.

The Structure

The best dynamic warm up sessions happen to be those that are structured optimally for the job. And in the remaining chapters of this book, we'll take a look at the different phases of an optimal dynamic warm up, i.e., the dynamic warm up structure, and how they all come together to ensure you have the most productive exercise and workout sessions each and every time.

Chapter 2

Self Myofascial Release

The first phase of an excellent dynamic warm up session is the Self Myofascial Release, or SMFR. This refers to hands-on technique that's effective and safe, which makes us of gently applied and sustained pressure. Such pressure is applied to the Myofascial connective tissue restriction to restore or even improve motion as well as to eliminate pain. You can minimize your risks for injuries and improve performance, function, and flexibility by using a piece of foam called a roller. Basically, you'll use your bodyweight by rolling on the foam roll in order to massage away normal soft tissue restrictions on flexibility and extensibility. The beautiful thing about this is that you can do this anytime and anywhere you are using a foam roller.

The Kinetic Chain

In order to fully understand how such a simple piece of un-high tech equipment can bring about such benefits and help you via a dynamic warm up, you must have a basic idea of something that's called the "kinetic chain". Basically, the kinetic chain is comprised several systems: the articular (joints), neural (central nervous system and nerves), and the soft tissue (fascia, ligaments, tendons, muscles) systems. Simply put, the kinetic chain functions like a tightly integrated functional group. Each and every component of this chain is interdependent with the others so if one of them isn't efficiently functioning, the other components will compensate for said inefficiency and in the process, overloading and fatiguing tissues. Over time, the effects of such overcompensation accumulate and lead to injuries.

A good way to look at this is to consider how restricted a particular joint's range of motion can be due to very tight muscles that surround it. Muscular restrictions such as neural-hyperactivity, soft tissue adhesions, and tightness can increase your risks for developing poor form and consequently, injuries. Through SMFR, you can address muscle restrictions, improve your joints' range of motion, and achieve much better muscular balance and physical performance.

Practicing Self Myofascial Release, especially as part of a dynamic warm up routine, has very specific benefits that can translate to much better exercise sessions, which include:

- Higher neuromuscular efficiency;
- Improved musculotendinous junction extensibility;

- Maintenance of normal length of functional muscles;

- Muscular imbalance correction;

- Reduced neuromuscular hyper tonicity, e.g., uncontrollable muscle spasms;

- Relief from joint stress and muscular soreness; and

- Wider range of motion for the joints.

In order to have a better appreciation for how SMFR works, it's important to know 2 important things: muscle fascia and trigger points.

Muscle Fascia

Fascia refers to a layer of specialized connective tissues that surround your joints, bones and muscles. These also provide protection and support to your body. This layer has 3 sub-layers namely the superficial, the deep, and the sub serous fasciae. Fascia can be considered as a type of dense connective tissue, which extends uninterrupted from your toes to the top of your head.

Many times, people think that fascia plays only a passive function, which is to transmit mechanical tension generated by outside forces or by the activity of the muscles. But lately, research has observed that fascia may also be able to contract smoothly as muscles do, which can influence the dynamic interaction of bones and muscles.

Trigger Points

Trigger points can be thought of as areas of the muscles that are painful and taut. Tissues can turn tough, thick, and knotted, and this can happen within muscles, tendon-muscle junctions, fat pads, or bursas. At times, inflammation accompanies trigger points and if the inflammation persists for an extended period of time, it can lead to inelastic scar tissue.

Speculations run about that many sports injuries are due to trigger points. These include anywhere from cramps to tendon and muscle tears. One plausible theory is that tissue structures are compromised by trigger points, which compel other tissues to make up for the compromise. Over time and with over-extended over-compensation, tissues can break down, which sets off a chain of undesirable consequences.

Many therapists believe that fascia trigger points have the ability to alter or restrict joint movement, which can lead to changes in the body's normal central nervous system function. Over time, these changes make the neuromuscular system less efficient, easily fatigued, chronically in pain, and frequently injured. These changes can also make a person's motor skill functions less efficient. If you're a competitive athlete, this is really bad news.

So why do trigger points form? There are several suspected causes, including inadequate rest and recovery in between exercise sessions, training too much, poor movement mechanics or posture, and acute physical traumas. And SMFR is a fairly simple method you can use to lighten or relieve trigger points. It's been shown in studies that Myofascial release can be effective in addressing Myofascial pain syndrome, albeit the studies focused on therapy-based Myofascial release rather than SMFR. Still, both work on the same principles and as such, it is reasonable to assume that SMFR can also be effective in addressing Myofascial pain syndrome.

General Guidelines

When doing Myofascial release all by yourself using a foam roller, you should ideally hold each position for up to 2 minutes per side, whenever applicable. But if you experience any pain, cease the rolling and stop where the pain is present. Rest on the painful area between 30 to 45 seconds. If you continue rolling despite the pain, you'll just increase that particular muscle's pain and tightness as rolling will activate that muscle's spindles.

When you stop the foam roller on the painful area and rest on it for up to 45 seconds, you'll inadvertently restrain the muscle spindles. This in turn reduces the tension in your muscle, leading to better regulation of the facial's receptors.

Choosing a Foam Roller

When buying a foam roller for SMFR, you'll need to consider the foam's density. Foam that's too soft will prevent you from experiencing an inadequate or substandard massage. Very hard foam on the other hand may make things worse, e.g., more pain, smaller range of motion, and inflammation due to greater soft-tissue trauma and bruising. That's why make sure you can give a particular foam roller a try first before checking it out at the sports store.

Specific Self-Myofascial Release Techniques

The IT Band SMFR

Lie on your side on a foam roll. You should raise your bottom leg slightly off the floor. Keep your head in a relatively neutral position where your shoulders and ears are aligned. Roll the foam just until below your hip joint along the side of your thigh down to your knee and back.

The Hamstring SMFR

Put your hamstrings (back of your thighs) on top of the foam roller, with the roller close to the back of your knee. Ensure your hips are unsupported. Cross your feet to maximize leverage and roll the foam up to the back of your hips (or your buttocks) and back. Keep your thighs tensed and tight all throughout the movement.

Thigh SMFR

Lie face down with your thighs resting on top of the foam roller. For this technique, you must ensure tight control over your core muscles, i.e., your abs must be drawn in and tight, and your butt muscles tight, so you can minimize or even prevent overcompensation by your lower back. Roll the foam to your pelvic bone, then to your knee and back.

The Lat SMFR

Lie on your side with your arm outstretched and the foam roller directly beneath your armpits. To ensure that your upper back – or lattisimus dorsi – muscles are pre-stretched for optimal release, point your thumb up. There is very little movement or rolling for this technique.

The Rhomboid SMFR

To clear your shoulder blades over your thoracic wall, cross your arms in front of your body to their respective opposite shoulders. Lie on your back with the foam roller beneath your rhomboid muscles, e.g., between your shoulder blades. Draw your abdominal muscles in keep them tight, raise your hips of the floor, and roll the foam to the middle back area and back.

Chapter 3

Mobility

The first phase – the self Myofascial release phase – was all about softening specific muscle tissues. In this phase, you'll be targeting those tissues using a combination of dynamic and short static stretching. The reason why we'll focus on short static stretches rather than long duration ones, i.e., 1 minute or more, is because the most recent studies have shown that long duration static stretches can actually be counterproductive – it can increase risks for injuries and lead to decreased physical performance during the exercise session itself.

Short duration static stretches will only take at most 30 seconds, which is considered to be appropriate for reducing excessive muscle tightness prior to the actual exercise session. This can help improve the quality of movement, particularly if there's a particular dysfunction in the muscles.

And of course, dynamic stretching will be the main star of this phase. It's because dynamic stretches – unlike static ones – require specific muscles and joints to move back and forth throughout their entire ranges of motion. This has the effect of "loosening" up muscles for optimal performance and lower injury risks during the main exercise sessions.

Dynamic Stretches

Twisting Lunges

This dynamic stretch combines two familiar moves – the forward lunge and of course, the torso twist. The lunge allows you to stretch your hip flexor muscles and in the process, activate your hip, glute, and leg muscles. The torso twist on the other hand, allows you to stretch your mid and upper back muscles, as well as helping you activate your core's rotation.

Perform a standard forward lunge but as you do, make sure your knees never go past your toes. Once in a lunge position, twist your torso towards the side of your lunging leg, i.e., right side if lunging with the right leg forward and vice versa. Do 10 reps and do the same with the other leg/side.

Knee-2-Chest

This dynamic stretch imitates the top portion of your running stride, where your knee moves toward the direction of your chest prior to your foot hitting the ground. Start by standing upright and alternately raise your knees to your chest as if doing an exaggerated march or walk in place. You can focus on closing the gap between your kneecap and your chest by pulling your shin in with each rep.

Elevation Kicks

These kicks will help you heat up your hammies and widen their range of motion. You can do this 2 ways: alternating (walking) and one leg at a time (stationary). Here's how to do it.

If you'll start with the right leg, extend your left hand and arm, and raise your right leg as high as you can until the toes touch your left palm. If you raise your left leg, extend your right hand/arm and touch that hand's palm with your left toes. Do about 10 reps for each leg per set.

Static Stretches

This one helps you loosen your chest muscles (pecs). Begin by standing upright with your feet just a bit wider than your shoulders. Bend your knees slightly and hold your arms out to the sides until they're parallel to the floor with your palms facing to the front. At this point, pull your hands as far back as you can to your back while keeping your arms straight. You'll feel a nice stretch on your chest muscles as you do this. Do 3 to 5 times holding it for a maximum of 30 seconds only.

<u>*Hammie Stretch*</u>

This stretch is for your hamstring muscles, a.k.a., your hammies. Start by sitting on the floor with both your legs extended and straight in front of you. Bend your right leg and let the sole of your right foot press along the inside of your left leg. Let your right leg relax on the floor and keeping your lower back straight all throughout, bend forward and try to reach as far as you can for your left foot's toes. Hold the position for at most 30 seconds, feeling a nice stretch on your hamstrings. Do the same for the right leg.

<u>*Calf Stretch*</u>

Stand upright 2 to 3 feet in front of a wall or a sturdy post. Start by stretching your left leg first. With both feet planted firmly on the floor and your body straight from head to toe, lean forward and plant both hands on the wall or on the post for support. Then, lift your right foot and take a step forward until your right toe touches the wall or is aligned with the post. With your left foot still firmly planted behind you, lean further forward until your right shin is perpendicular to the floor. At this point, you'll feel a nice stretch on your left calf muscle. Hold the position for no more than 30 seconds before switching to the right leg.

Chapter 4

Corrective Exercise

After you're done with the mobility phase of your dynamic warm up session, it's time to ensure that your overall movement system's efficient through the use of corrective exercises. These are exercises that are specifically programmed to address specific faulty patterns of movement that may affect your exercise performance or lead to injuries in the long run. And when it comes to corrective exercises, the cardinal rule is proper execution. In other words, you'll need to pay very close attention on each and every repetition to ensure proper form each time.

The reason for this lies in its primary purpose: correcting faulty movement patterns or habits. And doing this isn't just a physical issue – it's also mental. It will require changing your subconscious thinking about how to execute certain movements, particularly the faulty ones. If you don't, you run the risk of injuries over time.

Sample Exercises

Quad-Way Band Walk

This particular exercise helps correct any faulty movements involving your butt muscles and helps minimize your risks for knee injuries. A particular faulty movement that many athletes aren't aware of that can cause injuries is the "valgus", i.e., the knees move inward during jumping, landing, or performing squats. This faulty movement pattern tends to put excessive stress on the ACL or anterior cruciate ligaments, putting them at high risk for injury.

To perform this exercise, you'll need an elastic exercise band. Wrap it around above both your knees and assume an athletic stance with your feet just a bit wider than shoulder width. Keep your knees slightly bent.

Then, take several side steps while keeping your toes pointed forward and your knees forced to maintain the open position. Take several side steps back to your original position. Do 2 sets of 10 reps/sets per side.

Always keep your knees bent and make sure your knees and feet move together. To help you visualize how it looks like, think of yourself as a sumo wrestler in the starting position and moving sideways in such a position.

Single Leg Quad Rockbacks

This is a good corrective exercise for tight hips as it forces your hip joints to handle more stress and become more mobile. To do this, start by going down on the floor on all fours. Stretch your left leg out to your side and plant your left foot as far as possible to the side. Keep your spine neutral, then bring your hips/butt as far back as possible until your lower back is no longer naturally arched. Go forward again and rock back and fourth for 7 more reps or rockbacks before doing the same with the right leg extended. Do 2 sets for each side.

The Wankle

For many athletes, mobility of the ankles is very important because these don't just absorb force but generate it as well. Ankles can also provide crucial feedback during movement for staying correctly aligned. Unfortunately, many of today's shoes tend to minimize motion of the ankles with some sports even requiring excessive mobility restriction by taping the ankles. And with poor ankle strength and alignment, injuries are highly likely to happen.

This corrective movement will help you improve mobility in your ankle's joints and in the process, optimize your exercise performance and minimize risks for ankle injuries. Begin by positioning one of your feet's toes 3 to 4 inches away from a wall and keep that foot firmly planted on the floor. The other foot should also be planted firmly but behind your body. Put both hands on the wall for support and stability.

Rock the knee of your foot closest to the wall forward and over your toes until it lightly touches the wall. Rock back to your original position to complete one repetition. Do 9 more reps before performing 10 reps with the other knee. Do 2 sets each.

Chapter 5:

Activation

By this phase of your dynamic warm up, it's time to turn on or activate the specific muscles you'll be exercising for the session. And while this is also a form of corrective exercise, activations focus more on the intensity and quality of the muscles' contractions rather than form. The more you can fire those sleeping or dormant muscles, the better you'll be able to execute much bigger exercise movements during your session.

Sample Exercises

<u>Single Leg Bridges</u>

This activates your butt muscles, which are heavily utilized during squats and deadlifts. Start by lying on the floor on your back, both of your knees bent with your feet planted flat on the floor. With your arms extended at the sides, raise one leg towards the ceiling and above your hip. Keep it straight and, while doing so, lift your hips off the floor and squeeze the butt muscle of the leg you're using to lift your hips. As soon as your hips are aligned to your ribs, bring your hips down until it just lightly taps the ground, at which point raise them up again until aligned with the ribs to keep continuous tension on that particular butt muscle. Do 2 sets of 10 reps for each butt or leg.

The Clam

This helps activate your – yet again – butt muscles. Begin by lying on the floor on your side. Bend your knees at 90 degrees. Wear a resistance band around both your legs at slightly above your knees. Let your head rest on your upper arm to maintain neck alignment.

With your hips stacked and heels together, rotate your hip to lift your knee and in effect, opening your "clamshell" as far as possible without rocking your body out of alignment. Gradually "close" the clam by slowly lowering your knee back to the starting position. Perform 2 sets of 10 reps for each butt or side.

Scapular Activation

This exercise helps activate a key group of back muscles – the lats, lower traps, and rhomboids. Start by hanging from an overhead bar with your hands at about shoulder width. Use an overhand grip. Use your abdominal muscles to minimize swinging while executing the movement.

With arms straight, try to shrug – i.e., bring your shoulders as close as you can to your ears – in order for you to bring your body down by about an inch or two. Then, pull together your shoulder blades and squeeze your lat muscles to reverse the movement and raise yourself by an inch or two. Hold the position on top – perfectly packing your shoulders in – for several seconds before repeating. Do 2 sets of up to 10 reps.

Chapter 6

Foundational Movement Patterns

After priming up the specific muscles via activation and the other earlier phases, it's time to go bigger performing basic foundational movement patterns. While these aren't the main exercises themselves, these mimic the movements involved in such exercises and provides a higher level of activation, loosening up, and warming up. The main or foundational movement patterns of the human body are the hip hinge, the squat, the upper-body push, the lunge, the loaded carry, and the upper-body pull.

You don't have to perform all of these movements during your warm ups because even if you just focus on a couple of these movements, you can experience significant improvements in your exercise performance.

Sample Exercises

Bodyweight Squats

Stand upright with both feet planted firmly on the ground at wider than shoulder width. Place your hands behind your head, lower back straight, and eyes looking straight ahead, lower your body until your thighs are perpendicular to the floor. Push back up to complete one rep. Perform 2 sets of 10 to 12 reps.

Throughout the movement, always keep your lower back straight and never let your knees go over your toes to minimize risks for lower back and knee injuries, respectively.

Bodyweight Pushups

Assume a plank position with your arms about shoulder width apart and extended. Your body should resemble a decline plank. Keeping your body straight, lower your chest close to touching the floor before pushing back up to the starting position. Do 2 sets of 10 to 12 reps each.

Lunges

Stand upright. Take a step forward with your right leg then lower your left knee until it's a few inches off the ground before pushing back up to the starting position. Do 2 sets of 10 to 12 reps for each leg. Remember to keep your back straight and never let your knees go over your toes to minimize risks for lower back and knee injuries.

Chapter 7

Central Nervous System Development

We've now come to the last phase of our dynamic warm up structure, which is all about preparing the body for explosive movements and revving up the central nervous system. The movements or exercises involved in this phase are the most explosive and dynamic within the dynamic warm up structure given these focus on global muscle recruitment and coordination.

But you may be asking, why the heck do you need to include the development of the central nervous system here? Why is the central nervous system so important? Simple – it's because in general, the nervous system's responsible for controlling the contraction and stimulation of muscles. If the body's neural impulses aren't efficient, we'd be hard-pressed to control our muscles' movements efficiently.

While it sounds as if training the central nervous system's rocket science, the truth is it isn't. In fact, it can be classified into just a few areas: throwing, jumping, and sprinting. The primary focus during this phase is on the amount of effort put into each movement. Training the central nervous system involves explosive movements that coordinate many different muscles together and as such, training the muscles to fatigue isn't the goal. If it were, then it wouldn't be part of a warm up structure, would it?

Sample Exercises

Many central nervous system development exercises are very familiar, as you probably did many of these exercises in school or as part of your summer league sports activities. These include jumping jacks, rapid knee ups (running in place), jumping as high as you can for several jumps, and sprints. Also included are combination of boxing jabs, crosses, and haymakers, such as those done in TaeBo classes.

Chapter 8

Examples of Dynamic Warm Ups

As we end this book, I'd like you to get an idea of how it all looks like when they come together. Because when you get a general picture of how all the 6 phases of the dynamic warm up structure come together, then it'll be easier for you to customize your own dynamic warm up. Allow me to end this book by giving your 3 examples of a complete dynamic warm up structure involving the 6 phases.

Example #1

- Phase 1 (Self Myofascial Release): Hamstring SMFR

- Phase 2 (Mobility): Twisting Lunges

- Phase 3 (Corrective Exercise): Quad-Way Band Walk

- Phase 4 (Activation): Single-Leg Bridges

- Phase 5 (Foundational Movement Patterns): Bodyweight Squats

- Phase 6 (Central Nervous System Development): Sprints

Example #2

- Phase 1 (Self Myofascial Release): Thigh SMFR

- Phase 2 (Mobility): Elevation Kicks and Calf Stretch

- Phase 3 (Corrective Exercise): Single Leg Quad Rockbacks

- Phase 4 (Activation): The Clam

- Phase 5 (Foundational Movement Patterns): Bodyweight Push Ups

- Phase 6 (Central Nervous System Development): Rapid Knee Ups

Example #3

- Phase 1 (Self Myofascial Release): Rhomboid SMFR

- Phase 2 (Mobility): Knee2Chests and Hammie Stretch

- Phase 3 (Corrective Exercise): Wankles

- Phase 4 (Activation): Scapular Activation

- Phase 5 (Foundational Movement Patterns): Lunges

- Phase 6 (Central Nervous System Development): Jumping Jacks

45

Conclusion

We've now come to the end of this road, I mean book. And I have to give it to you, that's a lot of information to take in and process. But if there's one thing I hope you'd take away from this book, it is that an excellently structured dynamic warm up session right before your main exercise sessions is an absolute must if you want to maximize your efforts' results. But of course, the more takeaways you have from this book, the happier I'd be.

Now that you've learned how a good dynamic warm up is structured, I strongly encourage you to apply what you learned as soon as possible. You don't have to do everything in one fell swoop. No, apply 2 to 3 lessons at a time until you come to a point that you've applied them all. Take baby steps and win many small victories that will ultimately add up to a huge one. The more you put any application of knowledge off, the higher your risk of not applying anything at all becomes.

It's my hope that this book was both informative and engaging for you. Again, many thanks for buying this book.

Finally, if you enjoyed this book then I'd like to ask you for a favor. Will you be kind enough to leave a review for this book on Amazon? It would be greatly appreciated! Thank you!

Don't forget to follow us on <u>Twitter</u>, <u>Facebook</u> & <u>Instagram</u> and visit our website <u>www.prosencefitness.com</u> to get empowered, educated and inspired to become the best version of yourself in life! You deserve it.